SOMATIC EXERCISES BEGINNER'S GUIDE:

Simple therapy exercises to manage anxiety, release trauma, reduce stress, and mind-body b balance in less than 15 minutes a day.

Sandra Madruga

Disclaimer
This book's content is solely intended for informative and educational purposes. Despite having taken every precaution to guarantee the content's correctness and completeness, the author disclaims all explicit and implied representations and warranties regarding the information's trustworthiness, completeness, or fitness for any specific purpose. The content is based on the author's personal knowledge and experience, and should not be used as a substitute for professional advice.

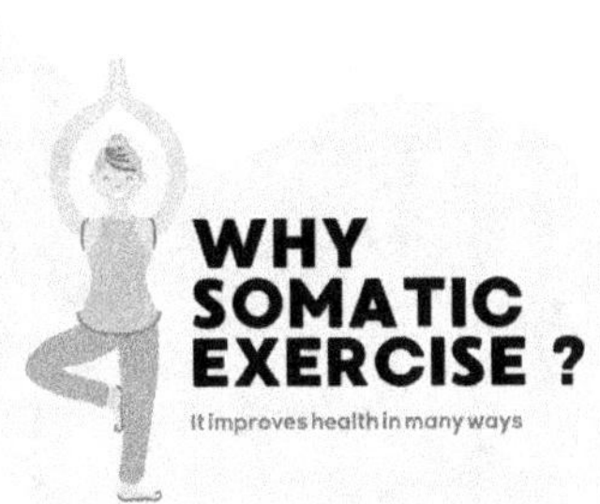

Improves Flexibility

Yoga increases your range of motion by stretching and moving your body in new ways.

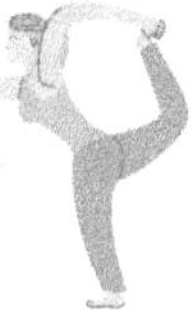

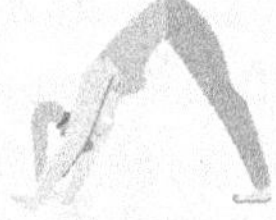

Reduces Stress

Yoga helps reduce stress and anxiety by encouraging mental and physical relaxation.

Promotes Better Sleep

Yoga promotes restful sleep by calming and relaxing the body after a stressful day.

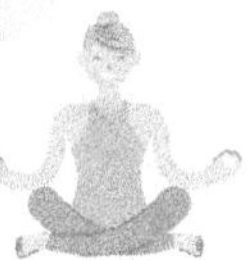

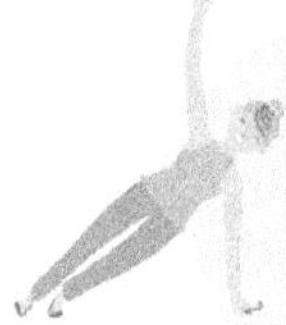

Builds Strength

The regular practice of yoga can help build lean muscle and improve strength.

Table Of Contents

Part I: Foundation.

Chapter 1: Understanding The Exercise.

Chapter 2: Getting Started

Chapter 3: Basic Exercises

Part II: Developing The Practice

Chapter 4: Intermediate Somatic Practices

Chapter 5: Advanced Somatic Techniques

Part III: Healing and Integration

Chapter 6: Understanding Trauma and the Body

Chapter 7: Exercises for Trauma Recovery

Chapter 8: Mind-Body Connection in Somatic Practice

Part IV: Integrating The Exercises into Daily Life

Chapter 9: Incorporating The Exercises into Daily Life

Chapter 10: Addressing Chronic Stress

Chapter 11 : Daily & Weekly Exercise Plan

-Final Notes

-Final Thoughts

Attitude Survey

It's critical to evaluate your present perspective and strategy in order to assist you on your path to stress management and improved wellbeing.

Give a sincere response to every question to learn more about your present methods and potential improvement areas.

1. How do you typically respond to stress?

- A) I react emotionally and feel overwhelmed.

- B) I try to manage it through quick fixes or distractions.
- C) I approach it with mindfulness and seek constructive solutions.

2. How often do you incorporate somatic practices into your daily routine?

- A) Rarely or never.
- B) Occasionally, but inconsistently.
- C) Regularly, as a key part of my daily routine.

3. How do you feel about setting realistic goals for stress management?

- A) I find it challenging and often set goals that are too ambitious.
- B) I set some goals, but they are not always practical or achievable.
- C) I set specific, realistic goals and follow a structured plan.

4. How would you describe your level of self-compassion?

- A) I am often critical of myself and find it hard to show compassion.
- B) I am somewhat compassionate but sometimes struggle with self-criticism.
- C) I practice self-compassion regularly and treat myself with kindness.

5. How do you integrate social support into your stress management strategy?

- A) I rarely seek support from others.
- B) I seek support occasionally but often handle stress on my own.
- C) I actively build and maintain supportive relationships and seek help when needed.

6. How effective are your current strategies for managing chronic stress?

- A) They are not effective, and I often feel overwhelmed.
- B) They offer some relief, but I still struggle with stress regularly.

- C) They are effective, and I feel more balanced and in control.

7. How open are you to experimenting with new stress management techniques?

- A) I am resistant to change and prefer sticking with what I know.
- B) I am somewhat open but hesitant to try new methods.
- C) I am eager to explore and incorporate new techniques into my routine.

8. How often do you review and adjust your stress management strategies?

- A) I rarely review or adjust my strategies.
- B) I review occasionally but don't always make changes.
- C) I regularly assess and adjust my strategies to improve effectiveness.

9. How often do you practice mindfulness or meditation?

- A) Never
- B) Occasionally
- C) Regularly

10. How do you handle setbacks or challenges in your stress management efforts?

- A) I feel discouraged and often give up.
- B) I experience frustration but try to persist.
- C) I view them as learning opportunities and adjust my approach.

Part I: Foundation.

Chapter 1: Understanding The Exercise.

A type of movement therapy called somatic exercises places an emphasis on an individual's interior bodily experience and perception. Somatic exercises place a higher priority on awareness of body sensations, movement patterns, and the relationship between mind and body than typical fitness regimens, which are more concerned with outward performance and appearance.

The objective is to promote a greater awareness and control of one's motions in order to enhance general well-being.

Benefits of Somatic Exercises

Numerous advantages of this workout improve emotional and physical health. Here are a few benefits:

Reduction of Stress
Somatic activities help people relax by fostering mindfulness and an awareness of their own body's sensations. This technique has a relaxing impact on the body and mind by easing physical tension and stress.

Enhanced alignment and posture

Somatic exercises can improve alignment and posture by raising awareness of how the body moves and feels. By encouraging more effective movement patterns, this advancement lowers the chance of injury and helps to avoid chronic pain.

Increased Mobility and Flexibility

In somatic exercises, the slow, deliberate motions improve mobility and flexibility. This enhancement facilitates a wider range of motion without strain, making daily tasks easier and more pleasant.

Pain Management

Somatic activities are quite effective in relieving chronic pain for many people. Pain can be reduced by concentrating on internal feelings and using light movement, especially in tense regions like the shoulders, back, and neck.

Mental Health

Somatic exercises emphasize the mind-body connection, which has the potential to improve emotional well-being. Enhancing one's feeling of equilibrium, anchoring, and centering via this technique helps boost one's mood and emotional fortitude.

Enhanced Mobility Effectiveness

Somatic exercises help people move in more conscious and efficient ways. This development can increase overall physical performance across a range of activities, resulting in more fluid and less physically demanding motions.

These advantages will be felt by you, resulting in a more integrated, balanced, and healthy feeling of well-being.

History and Evolution of Somatic Practices.

Somatic practices have a long history, having developed as a result of several advances in science and culture. These techniques are based on a profound awareness of the mind-body connection, feelings, and movements of the body.

The following highlights significant turning points in the development and history of somatic practices:

Old Roots

Ancient therapeutic traditions and ideologies, including the following, are the source of somatic practices:

1. Eastern Practices: Through deliberate movements, breathing exercises, and meditation, ancient Chinese and Indian practices like Tai Chi, Qigong, and Yoga highlight the unity of body and mind.

These practices, with their emphasis on balance and inward awareness, set the foundation for our current knowledge of somatics.

2. Western Traditions: The idea that the body is a living, sentient thing dates back to ancient Greece, where the concept of "somatics"

originated. The significance of holistic treatment was underscored by the exploration of the connection between physical and mental well-being by philosophers such as Hippocrates and Socrates.

Contemporary Expansion

Over the past few decades, somatic practices have been developing and becoming more diverse.

1. Body-Mind Centering: Created by Bonnie Bainbridge Cohen, this method focuses on developmental movement patterns and experiential anatomy to examine the connection between the mind and body.

2. Somatic Experiencing: By addressing the body's physiological reactions to stress, Dr. Peter Levine's approach focuses on trauma recovery. It has gained recognition for its effectiveness in

treating conditions related to trauma, including post-traumatic stress disorder (PTSD).

3. Integration with Modern Therapies: These days, somatic practices are increasingly integrated with modern therapeutic approaches, such as physical therapy, psychotherapy.

Chapter Overview

- You'll improve your physical and mental well-being, strengthen your relationship with your body, and feel better overall by including somatic exercises in your regimen.

- Originating in age-old customs, somatic practices have a long and varied history that is constantly changing due to advancements in science and creativity.

- This evolution offers useful tools for improving mental, emotional, and physical well-being and represents a growing knowledge of the intrinsic relationship between the body and mind.

Chapter 2: Getting Started

Setting Up a Safe Exercise Environment

A successful practice depends on creating the right environment. Here's a guide to help you set up a space that supports your journey:

1. Choosing the Right Space: Your practice area should be a quiet haven where you can focus undisturbed.

For instance, picture a comfortable corner of your living room with soft, natural light streaming through a window. You chose this spot because it's away from the household chaos; by shutting the door and turning off the TV, you've created a serene space dedicated to your practice.

2. Creating a Comfortable Atmosphere: The environment should be soothing and conducive to relaxation, creating the perfect environment for mindful practice.

For example, create a gentle glow in the room, arrange a few candles around it and use a dimmer switch to control the lighting. A soft wind from an open window wafts in the subtle aroma of lavender from a diffuser nearby. This arrangement aids in relaxation and mental preparation for your session.

3. Guaranteeing Accessibility and Safety

Note: There should be no risks present, and there should be a firm, non-slip surface for mobility.

For instance, you lay out a premium yoga mat on a spotless, flat surface. Make sure there are no furniture or stray objects in the way before you begin. You are able to move around the space safely and freely because there are no toys or loose wires that could cause you to trip.

4. Adding Comfort and Support

Comfort is key to a successful practice. Use props and wear appropriate clothing to enhance your experience.

As an illustration, you've set up a couple pillows and a cozy blanket for support. These cushions are positioned in strategic locations, such behind your knees or behind your lower back, to offer more comfort while performing stretches. You're wearing elastic, breathable gear that doesn't restrict your freedom of motion.

5. Getting Ready for Your Work

Being mentally and physically ready for a focused and productive session is part of preparation.

To keep hydrated, have a glass of water before you begin. Set a good intention for your practice by taking a minute to sit quietly and breathe deeply. Maybe you want to concentrate on letting go and unwinding, directing your mind to remain focused and in the moment during the session.

Essential Equipment and Attire

It doesn't need a lot of pricey equipment to set up a somatic exercise routine. You can set up a cozy and productive area for your workouts with a few essentials. This is a list of necessary, tested, and reasonably priced tools and clothing, along with real-world examples.

Essential Tools

1. A workout mat

An exercise mat is an essential piece of equipment for activities performed on the floor since it offers support and cushioning.

When I started my somatic journey, I discovered how important a good yoga mat was. I selected a thick, non-slip mat that offered my back and knees plenty of comfort while I stretched. There are plenty of reasonably priced mats on the market, and even a simple model may greatly improve stability and comfort.

2. Yoga Blocks: Yoga blocks are adaptable props that help with alignment and offer support for a range of positions.

Using yoga blocks improved my alignment and balance during the movements. For example, I used a block beneath my hands to assist my forward bends and increase my reach while I was doing mild stretching. Generally speaking, blocks are not costly.

3. A pillow or brace

More comfort and support may be obtained using a bolster or cushion, especially while doing sitting positions and relaxation techniques.

I found that for deep periods, a basic bolster or even a hard cushion was a great help for supporting my back. Usually lie on my back with the bolster under my knees to relieve tightness in my lower back. These products are frequently reasonably priced.

4. Resistance Bands

Resistance bands are a great way to strengthen muscles, improve flexibility, and add a little resistance to your activities.

I have resistance bands among my tools. I focused on conscious movement while using them to strengthen my muscles and do gentle stretches. Budget-friendly resistance bands are available in a range of resistance levels to meet diverse requirements.

Required Clothing

1. Cozy attire

You may move freely and without being constrained if you wear clothing that is breathable and flexible.

I began out with a comfy, moisture-wicking shirt and a pair of elastic yoga trousers. I felt free to move in a variety of ways while wearing these clothes. Numerous stores have reasonably priced athletic wear, and selecting things with breathable fabrics can keep you comfortable during your practice.

2. Bare feet or Non-slip socks

During workouts, wearing non-slip socks or being barefoot helps improve grip and stability.

I learned, among other things, that training on her mat with non-slip socks or bare feet offered superior traction. Especially while doing standing or balance-focused activities, this small adjustment helped me keep my balance and prevent slipping. Non-slip socks come in a variety of sports and department stores and are reasonably priced.

Chapter Overview

- You'll discover, as I did, that these simple tools really improve your practice and make it simpler to concentrate on your motions and meet your wellbeing objectives.

- You can make your somatic exercises practical and comfortable by choosing these key, well-proven, and reasonably priced pieces of gear and clothing.

Chapter 3: Basic Exercises

Breathing Techniques

An essential component of somatic workouts, these methods aid in stress reduction, anxiety management, and general wellbeing enhancement. These breathing exercises can help you get started.

Belly breathing, or Diaphragmatic breathing

Instead of inhaling shallowly from the chest, this calls for deep breathing from the diaphragm. This method encourages effective oxygen exchange and relaxation.

Step 1: Locate a Comfortable Position: Take a seat or lie down where you feel comfortable. Grasp your belly with one hand and your chest with the other.

2. Take a Deep Breath: - To begin this exercise, I took a deep breath through my nose and felt my belly rise as I filled my lungs with air. As long as my chest stays reasonably still, I'm using my diaphragm appropriately. For the guarantee of diaphragm usage, follow suit as well.

3. gently Exhale: - I also felt my abdomen drop as I gently breathed through my lips. To encourage relaxation, I made sure my exhale was longer than my inhale.

For five to ten minutes, keep up this deep breathing rhythm while paying attention to your abdomen's rise and fall.

4-7-8 Inhalation

This is a basic breathing technique that lowers tension and soothes the neurological system.

Step 1: Choose a Comfortable Position: Prop your back straight whether sitting or lying down.

2. Inhale: Shut your eyes and take a gentle, four-count inhalation via your nostrils.

3. Hold: Take a five-count breath hold.

4. Exhale: For a count of eight, let out all of your breath through your mouth while whooshing.

This cycle should be repeated four times. It's beneficial in the same way that I discovered this method to be quite helpful in helping her relax and get ready for bed.

Box breathing

This method helps to quiet the body and concentrate the mind. Although athletes employ this strategy frequently, it's also beneficial for highly pressured workers.

1. As always, choose a comfortable position. You can either lie down comfortably or sit up straight in a chair with your feet flat on the floor.

2. Inhale: Take a leisurely, four-count breath through your nose.

3. Hold: Take a seven-count breath hold.

4. Exhale: Take a leisurely, five-count breath out through your mouth.

5. Hold: Take another five deep breaths.

Remember to do this cycle five times. I frequently employ this strategy to help me stay composed and focused before big meetings.

Differential Nostril Inhalation

This method fosters a sense of peace and wellbeing by bringing the body and mind into harmony.

Step 1: Choose a Comfortable Position: Sit upright in a comfortable position.

2. Hand Position: Shut your right nostril with your thumb.

3. Inhale: Take a deep breath in through your left nose.

4. Switch: Using your right ring finger, close your left nostril and release your right.

5. Release the air through your right nostril, gently.

6. Inhale: Take a deep breath in through your right nose.

7. Switch and Exhale: Let go of your left nostril and close your right nose with your thumb. Breathe out slowly using your left nostril.

Do this for five to fifteen minutes at a time. Use this method to improve mental clarity and energy balance.

Resonant Breathing

By using this approach, you'll enhance heart rate variability and lower anxiety by breathing at a pace of five to six breaths per minute.

Steps
1: Choose a Comfortable Position: Take a seat or lie down.

2. Inhale: Take a five-count breath through your nose.

3. Exhale: Take a five-count breath out through your nose.

Repeat this sequence often while keeping a constant cadence. To maintain a steady pace, you might set a 10-minute timer.

You'll discover, as I did, that using these methods on a daily basis results in a more balanced body and calmer mind.

Progressive Relaxation.

This method entails tensing and then gradually releasing the body's various muscle groups. This technique encourages general relaxation by lowering tension and anxiety.

Getting Ready

-Find a Quiet Place: Decide on a peaceful, comfortable area free from interruptions. You have the option of lying on a yoga mat on the floor, in a chair, or on a bed.

- Become Comfortable: Take off any constricting items and dress in loose, cozy attire. Make sure your body has enough support.

After preparing, I essentially use gradual relaxation, winding down after a long day by doing the following:

1. Take a deep breath at first.

To begin, inhale deeply with your nose and exhale gently through your lips for a few deep breaths. This helps to center yourself and prepare for relaxation.

2. Concentrate on Every Muscle Group

Head and Face: Lift your eyebrows as high as you can to start tightening the muscles in your forehead. Maintain the strain for around five seconds.

Then let go of the tension, allowing your forehead to fully relax, and observe the distinction between the two states. After taking a ten-second break, go to the next muscle group.

Jaw: Tighten your jaw for a duration of five seconds.

Next, let go of the tightness in your jaw and concentrate on how relaxed you feel.

- Neck and Shoulders: Tension-build for five seconds by shrugging your shoulders up toward your ears.

After that, gradually drop your shoulders to release any tension. Your neck and shoulders will begin to relax.

- Arms and Hands: - Form a fist, bend the arms at the elbows, and hold the strain for five seconds to tighten the biceps.

Next, let go of the tension and fully relax your hands and arms.

-Abdomen and Chest: Tense the muscles in your abdomen and chest for five seconds while taking a deep breath and holding it.
Next, slowly exhale to let go of the tension and feel your torso become more relaxed.

- Legs and Feet: Press your legs together and point your toes to tighten your thigh muscles. Hold this position for five seconds.   Then let go of the tension and fully relax your legs and feet.

3. Check for Persistent Tension
Once you've worked on all the muscle groups, take a time to assess your body for any residual tension. Like I did, breathe deeply and visualize relaxation spreading through your body, melting away any residual tension.

4. Take a deep breath to finish.

Take a few more deep breaths to round up your session. Breathe in deeply with your nose and out slowly through your mouth. Slowly open your eyes and savor the profound sense of calm that comes with it.

This method improves your somatic practice and leads you to a deeper level of relaxation.

Easy Stretching Exercises

Simple stretching exercises can help you become more flexible, relieve stress in your muscles, and generally feel better. The exercises includes:

Full-Body Stretching Routine

Preparation

It's always necessary to be prepared.

Warm yourself up gently at first to get your circulation circulating. This might be a light marching in place or a five-minute walk.

-Make sure you have adequate room to move about. For increased comfort, consider using a yoga mat.
It's always necessary to be prepared.

Warm yourself up gently at first to get your circulation circulating. This might be a light marching in place or a five-minute walk.

-Make sure you have adequate room to move about. For increased comfort, consider using a yoga mat.

1. Stretch your neck

Steps:
  - Take a comfortable seat or stand with a straight back.

Extend:Start by turning your head slightly to the right and bringing your ear close to your shoulder. You should feel a slight stretch along the left side of your neck after holding the pose for 20 to 25 seconds.

- then makes a circle back to the center, repeating on the opposite side.

- Gently lay your palm on the side of your head and press a little bit to deepen the stretch.

2. Extension of the Shoulders

Steps: Sit or stand with a straight back.
-Subsequently, extend your right arm shoulder-high across your body. Hold the stretch for 15 to 20 seconds while using your left hand to gently push your right arm toward your chest.

3. Stretching the Upper Back

Steps: Ensure that you sit or stand with a straight back.

- Extend your arms in front of you to shoulder height while putting your hands together. You should feel a stretch between your shoulder blades as you round your upper back and gently push your hands away from your body.

-Holds the stretch for ten to fifteen seconds.

4. Stretching the chest

Procedure: - Place your feet shoulder-width apart. Next, extend your arms straight and interlace your fingers behind your back. Feel a stretch across your chest as you slowly raise your hands toward the sky while maintaining your shoulders down.

-Stretch for a duration of 15 to 20 seconds.

5. Bending to the side

Steps: Spread your feet shoulder-width apart as you stand.

- Feel the right half of your body expand as you raise your right arm aloft and sag slightly to the left.

-Stretches for 15 to 20 seconds, then alternates sides.

6. Stretching the Hamstrings

Steps: Take a seat on the ground and extend your legs straight in front of you.

-Keep your back straight as you extend your hand toward your toes.

-You should feel a stretch in the back of your legs after holding the pose for 15 to 20 seconds.

You can use a towel or yoga strap to help if you are unable to reach your toes.

7. Stretching the Quadriceps

Steps: To maintain balance, stand with your feet together and grasp a wall or chair.

-Bring your heel up to your buttocks and bend your right knee. Feel a stretch at the front of your thigh as you gently pull on your ankle with your right hand.
-20–25 seconds are spent holding the stretch.

8. Flex Your Calf

Steps: - Place your hands shoulder-height against the wall as you face it. Retrace your right foot while maintaining a straight leg and your heel on the ground. She feels a stretch in your right calf as she presses against the wall with her bent left knee.

9. Flexor Hammitors

Steps: Make a 90-degree angle at both knees by kneeling on the floor with your right knee on the floor and your left foot in front.
- Feel a stretch in the front of your right hip as you gently press your hips forward while maintaining a straight back.

You'll discover, all in all, that stretching on a daily basis promotes bodily balance and relaxation.

Chapter Summary

- You'll increase your general somatic well-being, decrease muscular tension, and increase your flexibility by including basic stretching techniques into your daily practice.

- By including breathing exercises into your everyday routine, you may manage stress, advance your somatic practice, and boost your general health.

- By incorporating progressive relaxation into your routine, you can manage stress more effectively, reduce anxiety, and improve your overall well-being.

Part II: Developing The Practice

Chapter 4: Intermediate Somatic Practices

<u>Pelvic Floor Exercises</u>

The muscles involved in this exercise are those at the base of the pelvis. These muscles support the intestines, the bladder, and the uterus in women. Maintaining the appropriate function of these organs depends on a robust pelvic floor, which is also essential for general core stability.

Benefits for Pelvic floor exercises

1. Better Bladder Control: Reducing urine incontinence can be achieved by strengthening the pelvic floor muscles.

2. Improved Sexual Health: Improved sexual performance and enjoyment can be attributed to stronger pelvic floor muscles.

3. Support During Pregnancy and Postpartum Recovery: These exercises are especially helpful for women to prevent and treat pelvic floor problems before, during, and after pregnancy.

4. Improved Core Strength: Exercises targeting the pelvic floor help to strengthen the core generally, which can help with back discomfort and posture.

Getting Started

It's crucial to identify your pelvic floor muscles before starting any activities. Urine can be stopped midstream as one method of doing this. Your pelvic floor muscles are what you employ for this.

Note: Because it might cause bladder problems, this procedure should only be used once to locate the muscles. As I did, I'll suggest it once a week. The workouts are:

Basic Exercises for the Pelvic Floor

☐ Kegel Exercises

Step 1: Find a comfortable spot to sit or lie down.
- Step 2: Contract your pelvic floor muscles and maintain that position for five counts.
- Step 3: Give your muscles a full five minutes of relaxation.
Step 4: Carry out this procedure five times.

☐ Combine Pelvic Floor Engagement with Bridge

- Step 1: Lay flat on your back with your feet hip-width apart and your knees bent.

- Step 2: Contract your muscles of the pelvic floor.

- Step 3: Raise your hips in the direction of the ceiling so that your shoulders and knees are in a straight line.

Step 4: Hold while maintaining the contraction of the pelvic floor muscles for a count of four.

- Step 5: Return your hips to the beginning posture while letting your muscles relax.

- Step 6: Five times over.

☐ Tilts in the Pelvis

- Step 1: Lay flat on your back with your feet flat on the ground and your knees bent.

- Step 2: Slightly tilt your pelvis forward while contracting your pelvic floor muscles.

- Step 3: Maintain the tilt for five counts.

- Step 4: Relax and return to the starting position.

- Step 5: Repeat 5 times.

Advanced Exercises for the Pelvic Floor

☐ Pelvic floor engagement during squats

Place your feet shoulder-width apart as your first step.

- Step 2: Contract your muscles of the pelvic floor.

- Step 3: Lower yourself into a squat while maintaining a straight back and your knees over your toes.

- Step 4: Maintain the squat while using your pelvic floor muscles for a count of five.

Step 5: Go back to your beginning posture and ease your tense muscles.

- Step 6: Five times over.

Core Strengthening Movements.

The muscles in the lower back, pelvis, and hips are also included in the core, in addition to the abdominal muscles. A robust core is necessary for:

i) Stability and Balance: It supports the spine and aids in maintaining good posture.
ii) Better Performance: In both everyday tasks and sports, core strength improves movement efficiency.
iii) Injury Prevention: By improving body alignment and support, a strong core lowers the chance of injuries.

Simple exercises to improve your core.

1. Board

- Step 1: Place your hands exactly under your shoulders and begin in the push-up posture, with your body in a straight line from your head to your heels.
- Step 2: Pull your belly button in the direction of your spine to activate your core muscles.

- Step 3: As your strength increases, progressively extend the time you spend in this posture by 15 to 25 seconds.

- Step 4: Maintain a steady breathing pattern while avoiding a sagging or elevated hip.

2. Dead Bug

- Step1: While lying on your back, bend your knees 90 degrees and stretch your arms toward the ceiling.

- Step 2: Press your lower back into the floor by using your core.

- Step 3: Slowly lower your right arm and left leg towards the floor while keeping your back flat.

- Step 4: Return to the starting position and repeat with the opposite arm and leg.

- Step 5: Perform 10-15 repetitions on each side.

3. The Bird Dog

- Step 1: on your hands and knees, placing your knees behind your hips and your wrists squarely beneath your shoulders.

Step 2: Maintaining a square posture at the hips and shoulders, extend your right arm forward and your left leg back.

- Step 3: Hold while using your core for a few seconds, then take a step back to the beginning.

- Step 4: Carry out step 4 on the other side.

Step 5: Work out five to ten reps on each side.

4. Bridge of Glute

- Step 1: Lay flat on your back with your feet hip-width apart and your knees bent.

Step 2: Form a straight line from your shoulders to your knees by using your core to elevate your hips toward the sky.

- Step 3: Squeeze your glutes at the top of the movement and hold for a few seconds.

- Step 4: Lower your hips back to the starting position.

Intermediate Exercises for Core Strengthening

1. Twists from Russia

- Step 1: Take a seat on the ground with your feet flat and your knees bent.
- Step 2: Hold a medicine ball or a weight with both hands and slant your back slightly while maintaining a straight spine.
- Step 3: Bring the weight next to your hip by using your core to twist your body to the right.
- Step 4: Go back to the center and do the left side again.

Step 5: Work each side for ten to fifteen repetitions.

2. Adjacent Plank

- Step 1: Arrange your legs straight while lying on your side, and support yourself with your elbow.
- Step 2: Raise your hips off the ground so that your feet and head are in a straight line.

- Step 3: Hold this position for 20-30 seconds, gradually increasing the time.

3. Lifting the Legs

- Step 1: Lay flat on your back with your arms at your sides and your legs straight.
Step 2: Lift your legs straight up toward the ceiling while using your core.
- Step 3: Lower your legs back down gradually, making sure they stay off the ground.
- Step 4: Repeat ten to fifteen times.

Advanced Exercises for Strengthening Your Core

1. Lifting Your Legs Up

- Step 1: Extend your arms fully while hanging from a pull-up bar.

Step 2: Lift your legs toward your chest while maintaining a straight or slightly bent posture by using your core.

Step 3: Return your legs to the beginning position slowly.

- Step 4: Repeat ten to fifteen times.

2. Bicycle Crunches

- Step 1: While lying on your back, raise your legs to a 90-degree angle and place your hands behind your head.

Step 2: Extend your right leg, engage your core, and move your right elbow toward your left knee.

Step 3: Exchange sides and move your left elbow up to your right knee.

- Step 4: Keep pedaling in an alternating side motion.

Step 5: Work each side for ten to fifteen repetitions.

3. Swiss Ball Rollouts

- Step 1: Place your forearms on a Swiss ball while kneeling on the ground.

Step 2: Roll the ball forward gently while stretching your body in a straight line by using your core.

Step 3: Return the ball to its initial location by rolling it.

Step 4: Complete five to ten repetitions.

Remember, consistent practice will lead to improved posture, better performance in physical activities, and a reduction in the risk of injuries.

Enhanced Flexibility.

Being flexible helps with improved posture, less chance of injury, and increased movement efficiency. It is an essential part of total fitness. Increasing adaptability can

- Expand Range of Motion: Enables more expansive and fluid motions.
Reduce Muscle Tension: This eases soreness and stiffness.
- Boost Circulation: Improving Muscle Blood Flow.
- Assist in Recovery: Promoting a quicker rate of muscle recovery following exercise.

Simple Flexibility Exercises

1. Hamstring stretches while standing

Place your feet hip-width apart as your first step.

Step 2: Stretch out your right leg forward, placing your toes pointed upward and your heel on the ground.

Step 3: Reach for your toes while bending at the hips and maintaining a straight back.

4. Hold the stretch for a duration of 20-30 seconds.

Step 5: Repeat while switching legs.

2. Stretching the quadriceps

- Step 1: Take a tall stance and use a chair or wall as a balancing aid.

- Step 2: Bring your heel up to your buttocks while bending your right knee.

- Step 3: Keep your knees close together as you grasp your right ankle with your right hand.

4. Hold the stretch for a duration of 20-30 seconds.

Step 5: Repeat while switching legs.

3. A chest opener

Place your feet shoulder-width apart as your first step.

- Step 2: Extend your arms and clasp your hands behind your back.

- Step 3: Squeeze your shoulder blades together, open your chest, and slightly raise your arms.

- Step 4: Release the stretch after holding it for 20 to 30 seconds.

Intermediate Flexibility Exercises

1. Forward Bend Seating

Step 1: Take a seat on the floor and extend your legs straight in front of you.

Step 2: Reach for your toes while bending at the hips and maintaining a straight back.

3. Hold the stretch for a duration of 20 to 30 seconds.

- Step 4: Go back to where you were before and do it again.

2. Stretching the hip flexors

- Tep 1: Form a 90-degree angle by bending at the right knee and placing your left foot in front.

- Step 2: Slightly bend forward to extend the front of your right hip.

3. Hold the stretch for a duration of 20 to 30 seconds.

3. The Cat-Cow Asymmetry

- Step 1: on your hands and knees, placing your knees behind your hips and your wrists squarely beneath your shoulders.

- Step 2: Take a breath, arch your back, and raise your tailbone and head toward the ceiling (Cow Pose).

Step 3: Let out a breath, arch your back, and bring your chin up to your chest (Cat Pose).

Advanced Exercises for Flexibility

1. The Pigeon Position

- Step 1: Begin on your hands and knees in a tabletop position.

Step 2: Extend your left leg straight back while bringing your right knee forward and placing it behind your right wrist.

- Step 3: Lower your hips toward the floor while bending your front leg and maintaining your rear leg straight.

4. Hold the stretch for a duration of 20-30 seconds.

Step 5: Repeat while switching legs.

2. Folding Forward While Standing

Place your feet hip-width apart as your first step.

- Step 2: Let your head and arms hang while bending at the hips and reaching toward the floor.

- Step 3: Return to a standing position gradually after holding the stretch for 20 to 30 seconds.

3. The Butterfly Extend

- Step 1: Place your feet together and bend your knees out to the sides while sitting on the floor.

- Step 2: Gently push your knees toward the floor while holding your feet with your hands.

- Step 3: Release the stretch after holding it for 20 to 30 seconds.

Chapter Overview

- Including pelvic floor exercises in your program can result in major gains in bladder control, core strength, and general wellbeing.

- By using these exercises for strengthening your core, you may develop a strong, steady, and well-balanced core.

- You'll enhance your overall physical performance and attain a wider range of motion and a decrease in muscular tension by consistently performing these flexibility exercises.

Chapter 5: Advanced Somatic Techniques

Somatic Yoga.

This blends somatic exercises with traditional yoga practices to improve general well-being, encourage relaxation, and increase body awareness. In order to reduce stress and increase range of motion, this method places a strong emphasis on deep breathing, gentle stretches, and mindful movement.

The advantages of somatic yoga

1. Enhanced Body Awareness: Encourages a closer relationship with your body so that you can identify and treat tense or uncomfortable regions.

2. tension Reduction: Utilizes deep breathing and relaxation methods to soothe the neurological system and lessen tension.

3. Enhanced Mobility and Flexibility: Mild exercises and stretches broaden your range of motion and flexibility.

4. Pain Relief: By reducing muscle tension and straightening posture, this technique can help reduce chronic pain and discomfort.

5. Emotional Healing: Promotes emotional health by assisting in the discharge of trauma and pent-up emotions.

Getting Started with Somatic Yoga

When starting a Somatic Yoga practice, choose a peaceful area where you may move freely and without interruptions. To assist with your practice, use a yoga mat or a cushioned surface. Dress comfortably and with room to move about.

Simple Somatic Yoga Pose

1. Cat-Cow Pose.

Steps
1. on your hands and knees, placing your knees beneath your hips and your wrists squarely beneath your shoulders.

- Step 2: Take a breath, arch your back, and raise your tailbone and head toward the ceiling (Cow Pose).

Step 3: Let out a breath, arch your back, and bring your chin up to your chest (Cat Pose).

- Step 4: Take five to ten calm, deliberate breaths while switching between these stances.

2. Child's Pose.

Steps

1. Spread your knees wide and bend your knees while knelt on the floor with your big toes touching.

   - Step 2: Lower your torso to the floor while sitting back on your heels and extending your arms forward.

   Step 3: Breathe deeply, letting your body relax as you rest your forehead on the mat.

   - Step 4: Breathe deeply and let go of any stress as you hold for one to three minutes.

3. The Supine Twist

Steps

1. Lay flat on your back with your feet flat on the ground and your knees bent.

   - Step 2: Form a T with your arms out to the sides.

   Step 3: Lower your knees to the right while maintaining a grounded posture.

Step 4: Shift your head to the left and hold it there for a minute or two, then alternate sides.

Intermediate Somatic Yoga Poses

1. The Bridge Position

Steps
1. Lay flat on your back with your feet hip-width apart and your knees bent.
   Step 2: Lift your hips toward the ceiling while pressing your feet into the mat.
   -Step 3: Press your arms into the mat and clasp your hands beneath your back.
   - Step 4: Lower your hips after releasing the hold after five to ten breaths.

2. Warrior II

Steps
1. Take a wide stance, bringing your left foot slightly in and your right foot out.

- Step 2: Extend your arms to the sides and bend your right knee such that it is over your right ankle.

- Step 3: Take a few deep breaths while gazing over your right hand. Then, switch sides.

3. Pigeon Pose - Step 1: Begin on your hands and knees in a tabletop position.

Step 2: Extend your left leg straight back while bringing your right knee forward and placing it behind your right wrist.

- Step 3: Lower your hips toward the floor while bending your front leg and maintaining your rear leg straight.

- Step 4: Exchange sides after holding for one to two minutes.

Proficient Somatic Yoga Pose

Pose with the Bound Angle Reclining

- Step 1: Lay flat on your back with your feet flat on the ground and your knees bent.

Step 2: Bend your knees to the sides and bring the soles of your feet together.

- Step 3: Rest your arms on your stomach or by your sides.

- Step 4: Hold for 2-5 minutes, focusing on deep, relaxed breathing.

2. Legs Up the Wall Pose: Step 1: Take a seat with your back to the wall.

- Step 2: Assume a reclined posture and raise your legs to the wall, bringing your hips in close proximity to the wall.

- Step 3: Breathe deeply while placing your arms at your sides.

- Step 4: Hold for five to ten minutes, letting your body fully decompress.

3. Sun Salutation (Corpse Pose)

- Step 1: Lay flat on your back with your arms at your sides and your legs out in front of you, palms up.

- Step 2: Shut your eyes and concentrate on your breathing while letting your body unwind fully.

- Step 3: Hold this position for five to ten minutes, or as long as you like.

Regular practice will help you achieve a balanced and harmonious mind-body experience.

Dynamic Movements

Exercises involving continuous, regulated, fluid motions are known as dynamic movements, and they are known to raise heart rate, improve circulation, and improve general body coordination. Dynamic movements added to your routine will:

- Boost Mobility: Increase your muscles' and joints' range of motion.
- Enhance Cardiovascular Health: Promote cardiovascular fitness by raising heart rate and blood flow.

- Get Ready for activity: Act as a useful warm-up to get the body ready for more strenuous activity.
- Encourage Functional Fitness: Boost the body's capacity to carry out daily tasks effectively.

Basic Dynamic Movements

1. Circles of arms

  - Step 1: Arrange your arms at shoulder height out to the sides while keeping your feet shoulder-width apart.
  - Step 2: Using your arms, draw little circles that progressively get bigger.
  - Step 3: Circle in one direction for thirty seconds, then the other way around.

2. Swings of the legs

  - Step 1: For support, stand close to a wall or other substantial object.
  - Step 2: Keep your right leg straight, swing it forth and backward.

Step 3: Swing for 15 to 20 counts, then switch legs and do it again.

3. Twists of Torso

Step1: Place your feet hip-width apart and bend your knees just a little bit.

- Step 2: Spread your arms out to the sides or place your hands on your hips.

- Step 3: Control Fully twist your torso to the left and then the right.

- Step 4: Twist each side 15 to 20 times.

Dynamic Movements in the Intermediate Level

1. Extensive Knees

Place your feet hip-width apart as your first step.

- Step 2: Quickly switch to lifting your left leg after lifting your right knee toward your chest.

- Step 3: Keep running for 30 to 60 seconds while rotating your knees.

2. Kicks to the butt

Place your feet hip-width apart as your first step.
- Step 2: While maintaining your pace, thrust your heels up toward your glutes.
- Step 3: Continue the motion for 30-60 seconds, maintaining a steady pace.

3. Twisting Lunges

Place your feet hip-width apart as your first step.
- Step 2: Step forward into a lunge, bending both knees to a 90-degree angle with your right leg.
walk 3: Turn your body to the right, walk back to the middle, and repeat from the beginning.
Step 4: Continue with the left side.
Step 5: Work each side for ten to fifteen repetitions.

More Complex Dynamic Motions

1. Leap Squats

Place your feet shoulder-width apart as your first step.

- Step 2: Lower yourself into a squat and then leap up with great force, raising your arms to the sky.

- Step 3: Softly land, then instantly return to a squat.

- Step 4: Repeat ten to fifteen times.

2. Mountain Climbers

- Step 1: Place your hands exactly beneath your shoulders to begin in the plank posture.

- Step 2: Quickly move to bring your left knee towards your chest after driving your right knee in that direction.

- Step 3: Keep running for 30 to 60 seconds while rotating your knees.

3. Jump Ropes

Place your feet shoulder-width apart as your first step.

- Step 2: Put your hands on the floor in front of you and lower yourself into a squat.

- Step 3: Reenter the plank posture by jumping your feet back.

- Step 4: Jump your feet back towards your hands after doing a push-up.

Step 5: Leap upward with a powerful leap, extending your arms upwards.

- Step 6: Repeat 10 to 15 times.

These exercises will serve as an effective warm-up or a standalone workout to enhance your overall physical well-being.

Integration with Everyday Activities.

Without requiring a separate, dedicated training time, including somatic exercises into your regular activities can help maintain and increase your physical and mental well-being. Throughout the day, this method guarantees that you maintain an active lifestyle, lower stress levels, and increase bodily awareness.

Morning Schedule

1. Morning Stretch - Step 1: Get up and raise your arms above your head as soon as you wake up.

   - Step 2: Lengthen your spine by stretching your body from your fingers to your toes.

   - Step 3: Breathe deeply while holding the stretch for 15 to 30 seconds.

2. Neck Rolls - Step 1: Maintain a straight back when sitting or standing.

   - Step 2: Slowly rotate your neck in a clockwise and counterclockwise direction.

   - Step 3: To relieve tension, roll five to ten times in each direction.

At Work

The first step in the seated cat-cow stretch is to sit at your desk with your feet flat on the ground.

Put your hands on your knees in step two.

- Step 3: Take a breath, raise your chest, and arch your back (Cow Pose).

Step 4: Release your breath, turn your back, and bring your chin up to your chest.

Step 5: Continue for five to ten breaths.

2. Chair Twist - First Step: Prop yourself up and place your feet flat on the ground.

- Step 2: Put your left hand on your right knee and your right hand on the back of the chair.

- Step 3: Turn your body to the right and cast an overhead glance.

- Step 4: Repeat by switching sides after holding for 15 to 30 seconds.

Leisure Time

1. Bending forward when standing

Place your feet hip-width apart as your first step.

Step 2: Reach for the floor while bending at the hips, allowing your arms and head to hang.

- Step 3: Return to a standing position gradually after holding for 15–30 seconds.

2. Push-ups against the wall

Step1: Take a position facing a wall that is roughly an arm's length away.

- Step 2: Spread your hands shoulder-width apart and place them on the wall.

- Step 3: Lean toward the wall with your elbows bent, then push yourself back to the starting position.

- Step 4: Repeat ten to fifteen times.

Evening Schedule

1. Legs Up the Wall Pose - First Step: Sit with your back to a wall.

- Step 2: Assume a reclined posture and raise your legs to the wall, bringing your hips in close proximity to the wall.

- Step 3: Breathe deeply while placing your arms at your sides.

- Step 4: Hold for five to ten minutes, letting your body fully decompress.

2. Reclining Bound Angle Pose - First, lie on your back with your feet flat on the floor and your knees bent.

Step 2: Bend your knees to the sides and bring the soles of your feet together.

- Step 3: Rest your arms on your stomach or by your sides.

- Step 4: Hold for 2-5 minutes, focusing on deep, relaxed breathing.

By making these small adjustments, you'll enjoy the benefits of improved body awareness, reduced stress, and enhanced overall fitness without the need for a separate workout session.

Chapter Overview

- Including Somatic Yoga in your practice will improve your general health by encouraging flexibility, calmness, and a closer relationship with your body.

- Adding dynamic movements to your training regimen will help you increase your functional fitness, cardiovascular health, and mobility.

- By including somatic exercises in your daily routine, you'll stay physically and mentally well even on your busiest days.

Part III: Healing and Integration

Chapter 6: Understanding Trauma and the Body

How Trauma Affects the Body.

Trauma is defined as a very upsetting or stressful event that exceeds a person's capacity for coping. This might be the consequence of repeated traumas like long-term abuse or neglect, or it can be the outcome of a single incident like an accident or assault. Trauma affects the body as well as the mind, showing itself in a variety of physiological and physical manifestations.

Physical Effects Of Trauma

1. Chronic muscular Tension - Because trauma keeps the body on high alert, it can cause chronic muscular tension. Pain, stiffness, and discomfort are frequently the outcomes of this strain, especially in the back, shoulders, and neck.

2. Modified Posture – People who have gone through trauma may take on defensive stances like slouching or hunching over. These shifts in posture have the potential to impact total body alignment and result in chronic musculoskeletal problems.

3. Increased Stress Response: Stress hormones like cortisol and adrenaline are released when trauma activates the body's stress response system. Prolonged stimulation of this system can

lead to hypertension, higher heart rate, and increased anxiety.

4. Digestive Problems - Trauma can cause abnormal digestion, which can result in symptoms including nausea, discomfort in the abdomen, and irritable bowel syndrome (IBS). Due to their effects on the gut-brain axis, stress and trauma frequently make these disorders worse.

5. Sleep Disturbances - People who have experienced trauma in the past may struggle to fall asleep, suffer nightmares, and have their sleep patterns disturbed. This may also have an effect on one's mental and physical wellbeing.

6. Immune System Suppression - Extended periods of stress and trauma can impair immunity, leaving people more prone to infections and diseases.

Hormonal and Neurological Effects

1. Modified Brain Function: Trauma can impact the amygdala, hippocampus, and prefrontal cortex, three brain regions that control emotions, memory, and stress reactions. Memory processing and emotional control issues may result from this.

2. Hormonal Imbalance: Prolonged trauma can throw off the equilibrium of hormones like cortisol and adrenaline, which are important in regulating stress. A continuous state of worry, despair, or emotional instability may be exacerbated by this imbalance.

3. Hypervigilance - People who are extremely sensitive to possible hazards may experience a prolonged state of heightened attention or hypervigilance. This condition may result in exhaustion, agitation, and trouble unwinding.

The Connection Between the Body and Mind

1. Somatic Experiencing: People who have experienced trauma frequently report feeling stiffness, numbness, or pain in certain bodily parts. The goal of somatic experience is to identify and treat these bodily signs of trauma.

2. Emotional Release: Unresolved trauma-related emotions may be stored in the body, which can cause emotional outbursts or chronic mood swings. Healing and emotional discharge can be facilitated by using somatic techniques to address these bodily experiences.

The Somatic Healing Science.

Somatic healing is the term for therapeutic approaches that address emotional and physical trauma by emphasizing the mind-body connection. This method makes use of the knowledge that emotional experiences are stored and processed by the body and that psychological as well as physical components of healing must be addressed.

95

Essential Ideas for Somatic Healing

1. Body Awareness: A key component of somatic healing is developing an awareness of one's own body's experiences. A greater awareness of one's body makes it easier to spot and treat tense or uncomfortable spots, which may be signs of unresolved emotional problems.

2. Mind-Body Connection: Somatic healing relies heavily on the mind-body connection. This idea recognizes that emotional and mental states have an impact on physical health and vice versa. Through addressing this relationship, people can experience recovery that is more comprehensive.

3. Trauma Storage: Studies reveal that the body may retain trauma as physical symptoms like pain or tense muscles. Theories like Peter Levine's Somatic Experiencing, which investigate how unresolved trauma impacts the

body's physiological reactions, lend credence to this idea.

Scientific Underpinnings of Physical Healing

1. Trauma's Neurobiology: Trauma has an impact on the nervous system and the brain. The hippocampus, which is involved in memory formation, and the amygdala, which regulates emotional reactions, are two important brain areas involved. These regions may change as a result of chronic trauma, impacting memory and emotional control.

2. Stress Response System: Traumatic events trigger the body's stress response system, which includes the hypothalamic-pituitary-adrenal (HPA) axis. Long-term stress can cause this system to become dysregulated, which can affect the levels of hormones like cortisol and adrenaline. Somatic activities aid in reestablishing equilibrium and controlling the stress response.

3. Stephen Porges developed the Polyvagal Theory, which describes how the autonomic nervous system controls physiological reactions to stress and trauma. This idea states that the vagus nerve is essential for controlling heart rhythm, digestion, and emotional reactions. The goal of somatic healing techniques is to activate the vagus nerve and encourage security and calmness.

4. Somatic Memory: According to the theory of somatic memory, the body retains memories of traumatic experiences. Tension patterns or bodily feelings may be the result of this storing. Body-focused treatments and movement exercises are examples of somatic practices that target these physical manifestations in order to promote emotional release and healing.

- For efficient healing and rehabilitation, one must comprehend the effects that trauma has on the body.

- The science behind somatic healing underscores the interconnectedness of the body and mind in processing and healing trauma.

- By understanding the physiological and neurological effects of trauma and employing somatic techniques, you can achieve a more comprehensive approach to healing that addresses both physical and emotional dimensions.

Chapter 7: Exercises for Trauma Recovery

Grounding Techniques.

The goal of grounding techniques is to assist people in reestablishing a connection with the present and their physical environment, particularly when they are dealing with stress, anxiety, or trauma. These methods can be particularly useful for controlling strong emotions and providing a feeling of security and stability.

Basicl Grounding Methods

1. The 5-4-3-2-1 Approach

- Step 1: List the five objects you can now see. Take note of the textures, colors, and details.
- Step 2: Take note of four senses. Feel the warmth of the sun, the feel of items on your feet, and the texture of the surroundings.
- Step 3: Pay attention to three distinct sounds. This sounds like rustling leaves, distant chatting, or the hum of a fan.
Step 4: Recognize two objects by scent. If you're indoors, concentrate on any smells in the space, or go outside to get some fresh air.
- Step 5: Take note of one flavor. This might be the flavor of food, a beverage, or even your own breath.

2. Body Scan

- Step 1: Take a seat or lie down where you feel comfortable.

- Step 2: To relax, close your eyes and take a few deep breaths.

- Step 3: Pay close attention to every area of your body, working your way up to your head from your toes.

- Step 4: Identify any tense or uncomfortable spots and deliberately release those muscles.

3. Grounding Through Touch

- Step 1: Take hold of a little item, such as a stress ball, a stone, or a piece of cloth.

- Step 2: Consider the object's warmth, weight, and texture.

- Step 3: Pay attention to your hand and finger feelings when you grasp or work with the object.

Intermediate Grounding Methods

1. Perceptual Experience

- Step 1: Go for a stroll outside while paying attention to how your body moves and how your feet feel on the earth.

- Step 2: Pay attention to the cadence of your strides and how your feet feel on various surfaces (such as concrete and grass).

2. Engaging The Senses

- Step 1: Select a sensory-engaging activity. Some examples include having a thoughtful shower, enjoying a warm beverage, or listening to relaxing music.

- Step 2: To ground oneself in the here and now, concentrate on the sensory aspects of the action, such as the taste, sound, or feel.

3. Visualization of a Safe Space

Step 1: Shut your eyes and picture yourself in a secure and cozy environment. This might be a hypothetical or actual location.

Step 2: Pay close attention to the intricacies of this area, such as the hues, patterns, and noises.

- Step 3: Allow yourself to feel at ease and safe by immersing yourself in this visualization for a few minutes.

Advanced Grounding Methods

1. Grounding Based on Movement

- Step 1: Take part in physical exercises that require awareness and movement, such tai chi, yoga, or stretching.
- Step 2: Pay attention to your body's motions and sensations. This will help you return to the present.

2. Conscious Inhalation

The first step is to choose a comfortable seat and lay one hand on your chest and the other on your belly.

Step 2: Breathe slowly and deeply while observing how your abdomen rises and falls and how air enters and exits your body.

Step 3: Keep going for a few minutes, focusing on your breathing and your sense of calm.

3. Getting in Touch with Nature

- Step 1: Go outside and spend time in a park, garden, or forest.

Step 2: Take note of the surrounding natural features, such as trees, water, and wildlife.

- Step 3: Notice how being in nature grounds you and allows you to sense a connection to the natural world.

You'll improve your mental health, promote stability in your life, and aid in your general healing process by implementing these activities into your daily routine.

Releasing Stress & Tension.

Stress and tension frequently build up in the body and mind, affecting general wellbeing. Maintaining health and improving quality of life require attending to these mental and physical states. Effectively releasing tension and handling stress may enhance mood, promote physical health, and enhance relaxation.

Creative Methods for Reducing Stress

1. Awareness of Somatic Breath.

- Step 1: Take a comfortable seat or lie down and let your body unwind.
- Step 2: Put your hands lightly on your belly while closing your eyes.
Step 3: Take a deep breath through your nose while feeling your belly expand and rise.
- Step 4: Gently exhale through your lips while paying attention to the feeling of release.
- Step 5: Keep practicing this concentrated breath awareness for ten to fifteen minutes, focusing on your tense spots while you breathe.

2. Intense Stretching Patterns

- Step 1: Begin with soft, flowing motions like leg swings or arm circles.

- Step 2: Include stretches for the main muscle groups as you gradually expand the range of motion.

- Step 3: Concentrate on breathing in time with your movements to improve your flexibility and level of relaxation.

- Step 4: Perform dynamic stretching for 10-15 minutes, allowing your body to release built-up tension.

3. Healing Touch Methods

- Step 1: Apply a little pressure with your fingertips to tense spots on your body, such as your neck or shoulders.

- Step 2: To encourage relaxation, use moderate kneading or circular strokes.

- Step 3: To further facilitate the release of tension, combine contact with deep breathing.

- Step 4: Practice therapeutic touch for five to ten minutes, concentrating on any tight or uncomfortable places.

Innovative Methods for Stress Management

1. Practices of Embodied Mindfulness

- Step 1: Take part in whole-body mindfulness exercises, such body-centered meditation or mindful walking.

Step 2: Become aware of your body's actions, sensations, and how it interacts with its surroundings.

Step 3: Engage in sensory sensations during your practice to help you stay anchored in the here and now for 15 to 20 minutes.

2. Interactive Relaxation Methods

- Step 1: Make use of guided meditations for relaxation applications with interactive features like guided imagery or biofeedback.

Step 2: Use the interactive tools to track and modify your relaxation reaction instantly.

- Step 3: Include these methods in your daily practice to improve stress management and self-awareness.

3. Expression and Movement of the Creative Mind

- Step 1: Investigate imaginative movement techniques, such expressive movement exercises or dance improvisation.
- Step 2: Let your body move naturally while concentrating on how your mental state is impacted by movement.
- Step 3: To process and let go of emotions, combine expressive hobbies like art or writing with movement.

You'll successfully handle both physical and mental strain by investigating and incorporating these cutting-edge strategies into your daily routine, which will promote a balanced and healthy lifestyle.

Techniques for Gentle Movement.

Techniques for gentle movement are useful tools for improving flexibility, encouraging relaxation, and bolstering general wellbeing. These techniques are especially helpful for those who are trying to manage their stress, get over trauma, or find a low-impact way to get healthier.

Guidelines for Practices of Gentle Movement

1. Mild Yoga

The purpose of gentle yoga is to increase flexibility and relaxation via slow, deliberate poses and movements.
- Basic Order:
1. Child's Pose: Lower your forehead to the mat while kneeling on the floor, sitting back on your heels, and extending your arms forward. Hold for a minute or two.

2. Legs-Up-the-Wall Pose: While lying on your back, stretch your legs out in front of you. Hold for ten to fifteen minutes.
Note: For support, use props like cushions or blocks. Keep your breath deep and your movements slow.

2. Karate

Deep breathing and slow, flowing motions are key components of the martial art of tai chi, which improves balance and calmness.
Basic Order:
1. Catch the Tail of the Bird: Step forward a little at first, using both hands to gently propel yourself forward. Five to ten times over.

2. Cloud Hands: Place your hands in a circular motion while shifting your weight from one foot to the other. Stand with your feet shoulder-width apart. Spend two to three minutes practicing.
3. dividing the Horse's Mane: To simulate dividing a horse's mane, step to one side and

extend one arm out and the other arm back. Five to ten repetitions for each side.

Proceed cautiously and at a moderate speed. Pay attention to deep breathing and smooth transitions.

3. Qian

Qigong cultivates energy and enhances health by combining breathing, movement, and meditation.

Basic Order:

1. The Brocade Eight: Execute eight actions, such as extending the arms and bending the body slightly. Spend a minute or two practicing each movement.

2. Five Animal Frolics: To encourage energy flow, mimic the motions of various animals, such tigers or cranes. For one to two minutes, mimic the actions of each animal.

3. The Tributaries of Treasures: As you move gently, visualize and concentrate on the body's

energy centers. Spend five to ten minutes practicing this.

Make fluid, flowing motions. Pay attention to your breathing and your mental imagery.

4. The Feldenkrais Method

Using slow, deliberate motions, this technique enhances body awareness and function.
- Fundamental Order:
1. Awareness Through Movement: Take a lying position and move your limbs and head in basic ways. Adhere to a scripted or guided session.
2. Functional Integration: To enhance coordination, practice particular motions, including getting up from a seated posture with little effort. For five to ten minutes, perform.

Move with awareness and curiosity. Avoid pushing yourself and focus on how each movement feels.

<u>**Chapter Overview**</u>

- Grounding techniques are valuable tools for managing stress and reconnecting with the present moment.

- Releasing tension and managing stress is essential for overall well-being.

Chapter 8: Mind-Body Connection in Somatic Practice

The Role of Mindfulness in Recovery.

Being mindful entails maintaining an open-minded, nonjudgmental mindset while paying close attention to the current moment. It is a technique that, through promoting awareness, acceptance, and emotional control, may greatly aid in the healing process following trauma and stress.

How Recovery Is Supported by Mindfulness

1. Strengthens the sense of self

People who practice mindfulness are encouraged to examine their ideas, emotions, and physical experiences objectively.

Enhanced self-awareness facilitates the identification and comprehension of emotional triggers and patterns, which can be vital in the management and resolution of symptoms associated with trauma.

2. Lessens Anxiety and Stress

The nervous system can be calmed with the use of mindfulness practices like meditation and attentive breathing.

People can feel more in control and stable by lowering their stress and anxiety levels by paying attention to the here and now.

3. Enhances Emotional Control

By teaching acceptance and non-reactivity to emotions, mindfulness enables people to notice their feelings without becoming overcome by them.

Better emotional control can lessen the severity of emotional swings and result in better reactions to stimuli.

4. Strengthens Resiliency

Through the promotion of an optimistic and adaptable mentality, regular mindfulness practice can increase resilience.

Those with more resilience are better able to handle obstacles and disappointments, which promotes a more well-rounded approach to rehabilitation.

5. Encourages Acceptance

Acceptance of one's current situation and experiences without seeking to alter them is facilitated by mindfulness.

Reducing internal conflict and resistance via acceptance of one's circumstances can result in a less stressful and more compassionate healing process.

You'll assist your path to recovery and wellbeing by including mindfulness exercises into your everyday routine.

<u>Meditation Practices.</u>

Meditation is a discipline that focuses the mind and develops a peaceful, clear mental state.

It has several advantages, such as lowered stress levels, better emotional control, and greater general wellbeing. People trying to manage chronic stress, anxiety, or trauma might benefit greatly from meditation methods.

Kinds of Mindfulness Practices

1. Meditation with mindfulness

The goal of mindfulness meditation is to develop present-moment awareness by paying attention to one's thoughts, feelings, and physical experiences.

- Fundamental Technique:

1. Take a comfortable seat with a straight back.

2. Shut your eyes and concentrate on your breathing.

3. Pay attention to how each breath in and breathe out feels.

4. If your thoughts stray, gently bring them back to your breathing.

5. Spend 10 to 20 minutes practicing.

It Enhances awareness, reduces stress, and improves emotional regulation.

2. Mindfulness with Loving-Kindness

Kindness and love In order to meditate, one must practice compassion and kindness toward both oneself and other people.

- Fundamental Technique:

1. Take a comfortable seat and shut your eyes.

2. Pay attention to yourself and mentally repeat affirmations such as "May I be happy" or "May I be healthy."

3. Gradually share these good vibes with family, friends, and even those you disagree with.

4. Spend ten to fifteen minutes practicing.

It increases sympathy, fosters happy emotions, and lessens feelings of loneliness.

3. Body Scan Meditation

Body scan meditation helps to develop body awareness and relieve physical stress by focusing attention on various body areas.

- Fundamentals:

1. Close your eyes while you lie down or take a comfortable seat.

2. Pay attention to every area of your body, working your way up from your toes.

3. Without passing judgment, take note of any feelings or tense spots.

4. Take ten to fifteen minutes to go over and unwind in each area.

It encourages relaxation, helps relieve physical tension, and heightens body awareness.

4. Guided Imagery

Using guided imagery, one can visualize peaceful and pleasant situations or memories to aid in relaxation and mental clarity.

- Basic Practice:

1. Take a comfortable seat or lie down, then close your eyes.

2. Either follow a script or listen to a tape of guided imagery.

3. Visualize yourself in a serene, unwinding setting, such a forest or beach.

4. Immerse yourself in the vision for ten to fifteen minutes.

It increases mental clarity, eases tension, and promotes relaxation.

5. Mindfulness-Based Transcendental

In order to achieve a profound level of relaxation and calm awareness, transcendental meditation practitioners recite a particular mantra.

- Fundamental Technique:

1. Take a comfortable seat and close your eyes.

2. Recite a mantra or word of your choice silently.

3. Permit the mantra's recitation to bring you serenity and concentration.

4. Spend fifteen to twenty minutes practicing.

It eases tension, encourages deep relaxation, and sharpens focus.

Chapter Overview

- Mindfulness plays a crucial role in the recovery process by enhancing self-awareness, reducing stress, and improving emotional regulation.

- By incorporating various meditative practices into your routine, you'll enhance your ability to manage stress, improve emotional well-being, and support overall health.

Part IV: Integrating The Exercises into Daily Life

Chapter 9: Incorporating The Exercises into Daily Life

<u>Short Routines for Busy Schedules.</u>

In the fast-paced world of today, it can be difficult to find time for exercise and self-care. On the other hand, adding quick somatic practices to your daily routine may aid in stress management, enhance your physical and mental health, and preserve a healthy mind-body connection.

These brief workouts are made to easily fit into even the busiest of schedules, so you can benefit without devoting a lot of time to them. Among these routines are:

1. Sun Salutation Sequence (2 Minutes) - Morning Energizer (5 Minutes):Practice a shortened version of the yoga sun salutation pose. This routine may enliven your body and mind with its flowing motions.

- One-minute Standing Side Stretch: Place your feet hip-width apart. Lean to the right and extend your left arm above your head to extend your body to the side, then hold for 30 seconds.

- Arm Circles (2 Minutes): Assume a tall stance and spread your arms outward. With your arms, slowly expand the little circles you make. To engage and release the shoulder muscles, perform this motion forward and backward for one minute each.

2. Reset at Midday (3 Minutes)

    - Seated Spinal Rotation: Take a seat comfortably, put your right hand on the chair's back, and rotate your torso to the right. This exercise takes one minute. After 30 seconds of holding, swap sides. This enhances spinal mobility and relieves back stress.

    Desk Push-Ups: Take a stance facing your desk, put your hands on the edge, and execute push-ups for one minute. This brief workout strengthens your upper body and increases blood flow.

    - Finger Stretch (1 Minute): Push your palms away from your body, extend your arms in front of you, and interlace your fingers. Shake out your hands after 30 seconds of holding in order to release any tension from writing or typing.

3. Evening Wind Down (5 Minutes): Sit or stand comfortably. Perform gentle neck stretches for

two minutes. Bring your ear to your shoulder as you slowly tilt your head to the right. After 30 seconds of holding, swap sides. Next, tilt your head slightly to gaze over each shoulder, pausing for half a minute on each side.

- One minute of ankle rotations: Sit with your feet flat on the ground. Elevate one foot off the floor and make circular movements with your ankle, moving in one direction at first and then the other. Repeat with the other ankle to relieve tension and improve circulation.

- 2 Minutes of Mindful Breathing: Take a comfortable seat and close your eyes. Pay attention to how you breathe: take a deep inhale with your nose, then release it gently through your mouth. Go on for another two minutes, giving your body and mind time to decompress and rest.

Somatic Practices in the Workplace.

The physical and mental strain that frequently results from spending extended amounts of time at a computer can be lessened by incorporating somatic activities into your job. These techniques are designed to be discrete and simple to follow without interfering with your job, encouraging improved posture, sharper attention, and general wellbeing. These workouts consist of:

1. Desk Ergonomics Check - Posture Adjustment: Make sure your feet are flat on the floor and that your chair supports your lower back. To avoid neck discomfort, place your computer screen at eye level.

2. Two minutes of seated shoulder and neck release
    - Neck Rolls: To relieve stress in your neck, slowly roll your head in a clockwise and counterclockwise circle for one minute.

- Shoulder Shrugs (1 Minute): Raise and then lower your shoulders in relation to your ears. To release tension in your shoulders, repeat this motion.

3. One-minute wrist and hand stretches

- Wrist Flexor Stretch: Raise one arm out in front of you, palm upward. Pull your fingers back toward your wrist with the other hand. After 30 seconds of holding, swap sides. This lessens the tension that comes with typing.

4. Twist While Seated (2 Minutes)

- Spinal Twist: Assume a straight posture, touch the back of your chair with your right hand, and rotate your upper body to the right. After a minute of holding, switch sides. This motion lessens back discomfort and preserves spinal flexibility.

5. 20-20-20 Eye Strain Relief (1 Minute) Rule: Take a 20-foot glance at anything for at least 20 seconds every 20 minutes. This lessens the

pressure that extended screen time puts on the eyes.

6. 2-Minute Breathing Break: 4-7-8 Breathing Technique: Take a comfortable seat and calmly inhale four times through your nose. After holding your breath for seven counts, let go entirely through your mouth for eight counts. Repeat for two minutes to help you focus better and feel less stressed.

7. Three-minute standing desk exercises

- Calf Raises (1 Minute): Using the balls of your feet as support, stand up and lift your heels off the floor. Return to the lower position and repeat. This strengthens and circulates blood better throughout your lower limbs.

- Hip Circles (1 Minute): While standing with your feet hip-width apart, move your hips in little circles. To relieve stress in your hips and lower back, perform this for 30 seconds in each direction.

- Forward Bend: Assume a standing position and extend your arms toward the floor while bending forward at the hips for one minute. Stretch your lower back and hamstrings by holding for a minute.

8. Micro-Meditation (2 Minutes)
- Mindfulness Pause: Close your eyes, take a few deep breaths, and focus on the present moment. Notice any sensations in your body or sounds around you. This brief pause can help reset your mind and improve concentration.

These somatic practices are easy to incorporate into your workday and can make a significant difference in how you feel both physically and mentally. Regular practice will lead to improved posture, reduced stress, and enhanced productivity.

Chapter 10: Addressing Chronic Stress

Understanding Chronic Stress.

If left untreated, chronic stress—a protracted and ongoing state of stress—can have detrimental effects on your health. Chronic stress lasts longer and might be more subtle than acute stress, which is transient and frequently linked to particular events.

Creating effective management solutions for chronic stress requires an understanding of its nature, causes, and effects on the body and mind.

Chronic Stress: What Is It?

A state of persistent physiological arousal is known as chronic stress. This happens when the body is exposed to stimuli frequently enough or intensely enough that the autonomic nervous system is unable to sufficiently trigger the relaxation response on a regular basis.

Causes Of Chronic Stress

1. Stress at Work: - Heavy workloads, tense deadlines, extended hours.
   - Unhappiness or insecurity at work.
   - Personal disputes with superiors or coworkers.

2. Stressors in Personal Life:
- Money problems.

- Issues with relationships.
- Duties related to providing care.

3. Environmental Stressors: – Residing in a dangerous or congested region.
- Being subjected to contaminated air or noise pollution.

4. The fourth category of lifestyle factors is poor nutrition and inactivity.
- Insufficient sleep.
- Overindulgence in social media and technology.

Physical Signs of Chronic Stress

Physical symptoms associated with chronic includes:
- Muscle Tension: Extended tenseness in the back, shoulders, and neck muscles in particular.

- Headaches: Often occurring migraines or tension headaches.

- Digestive Problems: diarrhea, constipation, bloating, or stomach discomfort.

- Cardiovascular Issues: elevated blood pressure, palpitations, or discomfort in the chest.

A weakened immune system makes one more vulnerable to diseases and infections.

motional and Mental Symptoms Of Chronic Stress

Chronic stress can have significant negative effects on the mind and emotions, which includes:
- Anxiety: A persistent state of anxiety and worry.
Depression: Depressing, despondent, and disinterested feelings in activities.
- Irritability: Enhanced annoyance and fury over little matters.

- Cognitive Difficulties: Issues with memory, focus, and making decisions.
- Burnout: A condition of extreme mental, emotional, and physical tiredness.

The Science Behind Stress and the Body

When faced with stress, the body undergoes a series of physiological changes called the "fight-or-flight" response. Stress hormones like cortisol and adrenaline are released in this process, priming the body to respond to an actual or imagined threat.

Although this reaction is beneficial in the short term, prolonged activation can have negative consequences on a number of body systems, such as:

1. Nervous System: Extended stress can result in an overactive sympathetic nervous system, which raises blood pressure, heart rate, and tension in the muscles.

2. Endocrine System: Prolonged stress can throw hormone balances off, which can have an impact on immunity, metabolism, and even reproductive health.

3. Cardiovascular System: Heart disease, hypertension, and other cardiovascular disorders can arise as a result of chronically elevated stress hormone levels.

4. Immune System: Prolonged stress can impair immunity, leaving the body more susceptible to illnesses and infections.

Effective management of chronic stress begins with an understanding of its nature and effects. You may lessen stress and enhance your general well-being by being aware of the warning signs and symptoms and acting accordingly.

The somatic methods and exercises that may be used to manage and reduce chronic stress will be discussed in the following section.

Methods for Stress Reduction.

Effective chronic stress management requires a variety of somatic therapies that address the body and mind. These methods are intended to improve body awareness, relieve long-standing stress, and encourage general relaxation. Here are a few somatic strategies that work well for managing long-term stress.

1. Flow of Somatic Movement

Gong Qi in Stress Reduction.
In order to nurture energy and lower stress, Qi Gong is an ancient Chinese technique that includes slow, deliberate movements, meditation, and breathing exercises.

Actions
1. Take a stance with your knees slightly bent and your feet shoulder-width apart.
2. Taking a deep breath, lift your arms to shoulder level with your hands facing downward.

3. Lower your arms and gently bend your knees as you release the breath slowly.

4. Repeat for 5-10 minutes, focusing on the flow of energy and your breath.

2. Activities for Sensory Awareness

Grounding Tactilely

The goal of this practice is to center oneself and de-stress through touch.

Actions

1. Take a comfortable seat with your hands resting on your thighs.

2. Carefully and slowly run your hands up and down your thighs, taking in the warmth of your flesh and the texture of your clothes.

3. Take note of the feelings beneath your fingertips and how they alter as you move.

3. Biomass energy

In order to alleviate tension and stress, this practice entails grounding through powerful, focused movements.

Actions

Place your feet shoulder-width apart as you stand.

2. With a strong exhale, lift one foot and stamp it down hard.

3. Continue for one to two minutes while repeating with the other foot.

4. 4. Focus on the sensation of your feet connecting with the ground and the release of energy with each stomp.

4. Body-Mind Integrative Techniques

Exercises for Releasing Tension and Trauma
        This entails a set of exercises meant to trigger the body's natural tremor response, which can aid in the release of deeply ingrained trauma and stress patterns in the muscles.

Actions

1. Lay flat on your back with your feet flat on the ground and your knees bent.

2. Raise your pelvis a little off the ground, then hold it there for a little while.

3. Allow your legs to tremble naturally as you slowly lower your pelvis.

4. Keep going for five to ten minutes, paying attention to the feelings that arise from the uncontrollable shaking.

5. Release of Dynamic Tension

Vibrating and Shaking

This method improves energy flow and relieves tension by shaking and vibrating the body.

Step 1: Assume a standing position with your feet shoulder-width apart.

2. Allow your body to naturally tremble as you begin by lightly bouncing on your heels.

3. Increase the intensity gradually while continuing to shake your arms, legs, and body.

4. After two to three minutes, slow down and observe the results.

6. Movement Integrated with Breath

Synced Breath-Based Stretching

Stretching and deep breathing are used in this exercise to improve body awareness and relaxation.

Actions
1. Take a comfortable position to stand or sit.
2. Exhale deeply as you raise your arms above your head and extend upward.
3. Bend forward at the hips and gently exhale, reaching for your toes.
4. Continue in cycles of five to ten, matching your breathing to the motion.

Including these somatic methods into your daily practice will provide fresh approaches to managing and lowering long-term stress. Every practice has different advantages that aid in stress relief, body awareness development, and relaxation.

Try out these methods to see which one suits you the most, then use them frequently for the best possible stress reduction.

Extended-Term Stress Management Techniques.

Implementing long-term methods that support persistent well-being is just as important to effective stress management as treating the symptoms when they arise.

These tactics center on developing resilience, leading a healthy lifestyle, and forming routines that facilitate continuous stress reduction. These are some long-term stress management techniques.

1. Create a Well-Balanced Schedule

Management of Daily Schedules

A daily routine that is planned and followed can reduce stress by bringing structure and predictability into one's life.

Actions

1. Establish time slots for work, exercise, eating, and unwinding.

2. Sort projects based on priority and divide them into doable portions.

3. Give yourself room to maneuver and modify your schedule as necessary to account for unforeseen circumstances.

2. Make self-care a priority

Frequent Exercise

Regular exercise can improve mood and lower stress hormones.

1. First, set a weekly goal of engaging in at least 150 minutes of moderate activity or 75 minutes of intense exercise.

2. Pick enjoyable hobbies, including dancing, cycling, or walking.

Optimal Eating Practices

A well-balanced diet can enhance your body's ability to withstand stress and promote general wellness.

1. Consume a range of nutrient-dense foods, such as whole grains, fruits, vegetables, lean meats, and veggies.
2. Drink plenty of water and cut back on alcohol and coffee.

Sufficient Sleep

Getting enough sleep is essential for managing stress and maintaining general health.

1. Aim for seven to nine hours of sleep every night.
2. Create a relaxing environment and stick to a regular sleep routine.
3. Gain Resilience Capabilities

Meditation and Mindfulness

Engaging in mindfulness techniques can improve your capacity to handle stress by encouraging awareness of the present moment and decreasing reactiveness.

Step 1: Engage in five to ten minutes of mindfulness meditation every day.

2. Practice mindfulness throughout the day to maintain your composure and sense of reality.

Thinking Positively and Being Kind to Yourself

Your reaction to stress can be enhanced by engaging in self-compassion exercises and developing a positive outlook.

Step 1: Counter negative ideas with affirmations that are upbeat.

2. Be nice and sympathetic to yourself, even when things are tough.

5. Prioritize and Set Realistic Objectives

Establishing Objectives and Managing Time

By avoiding overwhelm, setting realistic objectives and practicing good time management can help lower stress levels.

You will discover a detailed weekly and daily exercise schedule in the next chapter, which is intended to assist you in incorporating the exercises and methods we have covered. This program is designed to provide direction and structure as you start your fitness journey. It will provide you a precise plan to work within, which will make it simpler for you to incorporate the workouts into your routine.

As we go into the specific programs that will assist you in achieving a healthy mind-body connection, managing stress, and managing anxiety, stay tuned.

Actions

1. Establish SMART goals—specific, measurable, achievable, relevant, and time-bound.

2. Track assignments and keep track of progress by using time management tools, such digital applications or planners.

Acquire the Ability to Say No

Stress may be decreased and overcommitment can be avoided by learning to say no and set limits.

Actions

1. Evaluate your obligations and rank the things that are most crucial.

2. Gently turn down any more duties that might put you under too much stress.

6. Consistently Evaluate and Modify

Regular Self-Evaluation

Maintaining awareness of your stress levels and coping mechanisms will enable you to identify areas for improvement and stay on course.

Actions

1. Make time for introspection and evaluate your ability to cope with stress.

2. Modify your tactics as necessary to take into account any new stresses or life changes.

Long-term stress reduction techniques include establishing a healthy habit, placing a high value on self-care, being resilient, forming close social bonds, defining reasonable goals, and routinely evaluating your strategy.

You'll successfully manage stress and improve your general well-being by incorporating these tactics into your everyday life.

Chapter 11 : Daily & Weekly Exercise Plan

It's time to put everything you've learned about the different somatic exercises and fitness methods into practice. You can stay organized and motivated while you work toward your wellness and fitness objectives by creating daily and weekly plans.

Choose any exercise from the somatic practices we've covered in the chapters to begin your routine. You are free to combine and modify these workouts to fit your own requirements and preferences.

As always, consistency is essential. For optimal effects, include these techniques on a regular basis into your daily and weekly routine. As always, consistency is essential.

Day 1

Date:	Name:

Age:	Goals:

Legs(Somatic Awareness)

Exercises	Reps	Duration	Notes
Warm Up			
Gentle Stretching			
PMR			
Body Scan Meditation			
Walking Meditation			

Day 2

Date:	Name:

Age:	Goals:

Back & Shoulders (Breathing Techniques)

Exercises	Reps	Duration	Notes
Diaphragmatic breath			
Box Breathing			
4-7-8 Breathing			
ATB			

Day 3

Date:	Name:

Age:	Goals:

Chest (Core Connection)

Exercises	Reps	Duration	Notes
Plank with chest tap			
Push-up with knee tuck			
Chest-pres			

s with leg lifts			
Bicycle Crunches			

Day 4

Name:	Date:

Age:	Goals:

Biceps & Triceps (Somatic Stretching)

Exercises	Reps	Duration	Notes
Biceps curls			
Hammer			

Curls			
Triceps Dips			
Cat-Cow Stretch			

Day 5

Name:	Date:

Age:	Goals:

Cardio & Abs (Mind-Body Balance)

Exercises	Reps	Duration	Notes
Jumping Jacks			

Burpees			
Russian Twists			
TaiChi Slow Movement			

Day 6

Date:	Name:

Age:	Goals:

Flexibility (Somatic Integration)

Exercises	Reps	Duration	Notes
Seated Forward Fold			
Butterfly Stretch			
Somatic Flow Sequence			
Somatic stretch and release			

Day 7

Name:	Date:

Age:	Goals:

Rest and Recovery

Exercises	Reps	Duration	Notes
Legs Up The Wall			
Gentle Neck Stretches			
Deep Breathing With Visualizati on			
Self-Myof ascial Release			

    As you participate in these rest and recuperation techniques, keep in mind that relaxation is an integral aspect of your development rather than merely a break in your journey. Your mind and soul require times of quiet and attention, just as your muscles need time to repair and get stronger after a workout.

Treat yourself with kindness and devote the same amount of attention to your body's need for rest as you do to your busy endeavors.Every breath you take during these peaceful activities is a step toward improved well-being and inner serenity, and you are worthy of this care.

Take this time for yourself—it's an investment in your health, happiness, and holistic balance.

Final Note

As you begin your journey with this book, keep in mind that improving wellbeing and stress management are ongoing processes. Take Mary's case, a busy executive who formerly felt overburdened by her demanding work and personal responsibilities—my sister, to whom I taught these exercises. She made the decision to incorporate brief somatic exercises into her everyday regimen because she was often under stress.

She progressively introduced mindfulness meditation to her nights, began with only five minutes of deep breathing in the morning, and included quick stretching sessions throughout her work breaks. She eventually experienced more clarity, less anxiety, and better general health as a result of these routines. She discovered that she could more successfully manage stress and experience a stronger feeling of balance if she regularly used these tactics and modified them to match her circumstances.

Embrace each practice with patience and devotion, as Mary did, and give yourself the grace to adapt and grow. The actions you take now will set you on the path to long-term wellbeing.

Final Thoughts

I appreciate you coming along on this somatic and stress-reduction journey with me. With these realizations and methods, I hope you will be able to make long-lasting, constructive adjustments in your life. I'm impressed by your dedication to wellbeing and urge you to keep learning about and using these techniques.

If you felt this book was useful, please think about writing a review. Your comments not only encourage me in my work but also assist others in getting the support they require. Thank you for your support and dedication to a healthier, more balanced life.